MAKING SEX SWEETER THAN EVER

Reaching New Peaks Of Sexual Satisfaction After 40 For Men And Women

Dr. Fredrick Kim

TABLE OF CONTENTS

INTRODUCTION

Aging is a natural and beautiful part of life, bringing with it wisdom, experience, and, often, a deeper understanding of oneself. For many, the years after 40 mark a time of renewed focus on health, relationships, and personal fulfillment. This period also presents an opportunity to rediscover and enhance your sexual well-being.

Contrary to popular myths, sexual satisfaction does not diminish with age—it evolves. With changing hormones, shifts in energy levels, and a wealth of life experiences, intimacy can take on new and exciting dimensions. In fact, many people find that their sex lives become more meaningful, fulfilling, and adventurous as they embrace this phase of life.

This guide is designed to help you navigate the changes, address potential challenges, and unlock new heights of pleasure and intimacy. Whether you're looking to strengthen your connection with your partner, explore new dimensions of sensuality, or reignite your passion, the tools and strategies outlined here will empower you to make sex sweeter than ever.

So, let's redefine what it means to experience pleasure, intimacy, and connection after 40. With the right mindset and approach, this can be the most fulfilling chapter of your sexual journey.

CHAPTER 1
Understanding the Changes After 40

Hormonal Shifts and Their Impact on Libido

As you age, your body undergoes natural hormonal changes that can influence your sexual health and drive. For women, a decline in estrogen during perimenopause and menopause often leads to vaginal dryness, decreased elasticity, and shifts in arousal patterns. These changes can sometimes make sex uncomfortable if not addressed, but they also open opportunities to explore new forms of intimacy and self-care.

For men, lower testosterone levels may result in changes in libido, stamina, and erection quality. However, these shifts do not signal an end to sexual enjoyment. Instead, they encourage you to adapt and redefine what satisfying intimacy looks like for you and your partner.

Embracing Your Body's New Rhythm
Your body's responses may differ now compared to your younger years, but this doesn't mean less pleasure—it means discovering what works best for you at this stage. Slower arousal can lead to prolonged intimacy, giving both partners more time to explore and connect. By paying attention to how your body feels and responds, you can develop a deeper appreciation for your unique sensuality.

Focusing on Overall Health
Sexual wellness is deeply tied to overall health. As metabolism slows and energy levels fluctuate, staying active and maintaining a balanced diet can support sexual vitality. Conditions such as high blood pressure, diabetes, or hormonal imbalances may also affect libido or performance, making regular medical check-ups essential.

The Psychological Aspect of Sexuality
Beyond physical changes, emotional and psychological factors play a significant role in your sexual experience. Increased confidence, emotional maturity, and a stronger sense of self often accompany age, enabling you to approach intimacy with greater awareness and intention. For some, overcoming societal stigmas or personal insecurities about aging can be a powerful step toward rekindling passion.

Shifting Priorities and Redefining Pleasure
In your 40s and beyond, intimacy often becomes less about performance and more about connection, experimentation, and pleasure in its broadest sense. By focusing on mutual satisfaction and understanding, you can foster a richer and more fulfilling sexual relationship that aligns with this new chapter of life.

By understanding and embracing these changes, you'll be better equipped to approach your sexual wellness with confidence and curiosity, setting the stage for deeper satisfaction and connection.

CHAPTER 2
Effective Communication: The Key to Intimacy

Open and honest communication is the foundation of a healthy, satisfying sexual relationship, especially as needs and desires evolve with age. Discussing intimacy can feel vulnerable, but it's a powerful way to build trust, strengthen your emotional connection, and reignite passion.

The Importance of Talking About Sex

As life changes—whether due to aging, shifting priorities, or external stressors—sexual preferences, needs, and boundaries may also change. Honest discussions about these topics ensure both partners feel heard, respected, and valued. Open communication can help you:

Address concerns such as decreased libido or discomfort.

Share fantasies or desires to keep intimacy exciting.

Clarify misunderstandings about your partner's needs or actions.

Creating a Safe Space for Dialogue

Effective communication requires both partners to feel safe and free from judgment. To foster this environment:

Choose a relaxed setting for conversations, away from distractions or time pressure.

Use "I" statements to express your feelings and needs, such as, "I feel closer to you when we take time for intimacy."

Listen actively without interrupting, showing empathy and understanding.

Discussing Desires, Boundaries, and Fantasies

Talking about your sexual desires and boundaries can feel intimidating, but it's a crucial step toward deeper intimacy. Here's how to navigate these conversations:

Start with Positivity: Frame your desires in a positive light. For example, "I love when we try new things together—how about exploring [specific idea]?"

Be Open to Feedback: Encourage your partner to share their thoughts and feelings, and respond with understanding.

Respect Boundaries: If your partner expresses discomfort about an idea, honor their feelings and find mutual ground to explore.

Revisiting the Conversation

Sexual communication is not a one-time discussion— it's an ongoing dialogue that evolves over time. Regularly check in with your partner to discuss how things are going, share new thoughts, or address any concerns that arise.

Schedule time to talk when you're both relaxed and open, rather than during moments of stress or conflict.

Use these conversations to celebrate what's working well in your relationship and explore ways to enhance intimacy further.

The Role of Non-Verbal Communication

Not all communication needs words. Body language, touch, and shared experiences often speak volumes in a relationship. Paying attention to your partner's non-verbal cues can help you understand their desires and comfort levels during intimacy.

By prioritizing communication, you create a stronger foundation for intimacy, allowing both partners to feel seen, understood, and deeply connected. When you share openly and honestly, sex becomes not just a physical act but a meaningful expression of love and trust.

CHAPTER 3
The Power of Foreplay

Foreplay is often described as the prelude to intimacy, but in truth, it is an essential part of the sexual experience itself. As you age, foreplay becomes even more significant, not just for physical arousal but also for emotional connection and overall satisfaction. Taking the time to explore and enjoy foreplay can transform your intimacy, making sex sweeter, deeper, and more fulfilling.

Why Foreplay Becomes More Important After 40 Physiological Changes

For women, decreased estrogen levels can slow natural lubrication and arousal. Foreplay provides the time and stimulation needed for the body to prepare for penetration, ensuring comfort and pleasure.

For men, slower arousal can enhance the anticipation and emotional connection, making the overall experience more satisfying.

Emotional Bonding

Foreplay fosters a sense of closeness and intimacy that strengthens your emotional connection. The slower pace allows both partners to feel seen, cherished, and desired.

Heightened Pleasure

Building arousal gradually through foreplay can lead to more intense orgasms and heightened overall satisfaction.

Expanding Your Definition of Foreplay

Foreplay is more than just a warm-up; it's about exploring pleasure and connection in its many forms. Some ideas to expand your foreplay repertoire include:

Kissing and Caressing: Take your time with prolonged kissing, gentle touches, and exploring sensitive areas of the body.

Massage: Incorporate sensual massage with oils or lotions to relax each other and ignite physical connection.

Verbal Intimacy: Whispering sweet nothings, sharing fantasies, or simply expressing admiration can be incredibly arousing.

Playfulness: Introduce fun elements like games, roleplay, or teasing to build anticipation and excitement.

Exploring New Forms of Touch and Sensual Play

As your body changes, so might your erogenous zones. Use foreplay as an opportunity to rediscover what feels good:

Experiment with gentle touch, firm pressure, or different textures like feathers or silk.

Explore areas like the neck, ears, lower back, or inner thighs, which may be particularly responsive.

Incorporate temperature play using warm oils or cool objects for heightened sensation.

Making Time for Foreplay

Busy lives can make it easy to rush intimacy, but dedicating time to foreplay is essential for deepening connection and pleasure:

Schedule intimate evenings where you can focus solely on each other, free from distractions.
Treat foreplay as a journey, not a chore—let the process itself be as enjoyable as the destination.

Communicating During Foreplay

Talk to your partner about what feels good and be receptive to their feedback. Encourage open, non-judgmental communication to ensure both of you feel comfortable exploring new sensations.

Use verbal affirmations like "That feels amazing" to guide your partner.
Pay attention to non-verbal cues such as body language, breathing patterns, or vocal responses.

Foreplay is the art of building anticipation, connection, and pleasure. By embracing its power, you not only enhance the physical aspects of intimacy but also nurture the emotional bond that makes sex meaningful and extraordinary.

CHAPTER 4
Physical Health and Its Impact on Pleasure

Your physical health plays a vital role in your sexual well-being, especially as you age. A healthy body supports stamina, flexibility, and responsiveness, all of which contribute to a fulfilling sex life. By prioritizing fitness, nutrition, and wellness, you can enhance your sexual experience and maintain vitality well into your 40s and beyond.

The Role of Exercise in Sexual Wellness

Regular physical activity benefits not only your overall health but also your sexual satisfaction. Key ways exercise enhances sexual health include:

Improved Circulation: Cardio exercises, such as walking, running, or cycling, boost blood flow, which is essential for arousal and responsiveness in both men and women.

Increased Stamina: Strength training and aerobic activities enhance energy levels, allowing you to enjoy longer and more fulfilling intimate moments.

Flexibility and Strength: Exercises like yoga or pilates improve flexibility, core strength, and balance, which can make experimenting with different positions more comfortable and enjoyable.

Enhanced Hormonal Balance: Physical activity helps regulate hormones, potentially improving libido and mood.

Key Activities for Sexual Wellness:

Kegels: Strengthen pelvic floor muscles to enhance control and pleasure during sex.

Yoga: Increases body awareness, flexibility, and relaxation, promoting better intimacy.

Strength Training: Builds endurance and boosts testosterone levels, which can positively impact libido.

Nutrition and Its Effect on Libido
What you eat directly affects your energy, hormone production, and overall vitality. A balanced diet rich in nutrients can support sexual health by:

Boosting Circulation: Foods high in antioxidants (e.g., berries, leafy greens) and omega-3 fatty acids (e.g., salmon, walnuts) promote healthy blood flow.

Balancing Hormones: Nutrient-rich foods, such as lean proteins, whole grains, and healthy fats, support hormone production and regulation.

Increasing Energy Levels: Complex carbohydrates and iron-rich foods help combat fatigue, ensuring you have the stamina for intimacy.

Foods to Include:
Dark chocolate (promotes endorphin release and mood enhancement).
Oysters and zinc-rich foods (boost testosterone levels).
Nuts and seeds (improve blood flow and energy).

Managing Health Conditions That Affect Intimacy

Chronic health issues like high blood pressure, diabetes, or arthritis can impact sexual health. Addressing these conditions proactively can make a significant difference:

Work with your healthcare provider to manage symptoms effectively.

Explore adaptive approaches to intimacy that accommodate physical limitations, such as using pillows for support or experimenting with positions that reduce strain.

The Connection Between Mental and Physical Health

Stress, anxiety, and depression can take a toll on both physical and sexual health. Incorporating stress-reducing practices into your routine, such as mindfulness, meditation, or deep breathing, can improve overall well-being and enhance your ability to enjoy intimacy.

Prioritize good sleep hygiene, as fatigue can significantly impact libido.
Engage in activities that boost mood, such as hobbies, socializing, or spending time outdoors.

The Importance of Regular Check-Ups
Maintaining your sexual health requires regular medical check-ups. Hormonal imbalances, cardiovascular issues, or other medical conditions can subtly affect sexual performance and desire. By consulting with your doctor:

Identify any underlying issues that may impact your sexual health.
Discuss options such as hormone replacement therapy, medications, or supplements that could enhance your experience.

By investing in your physical health, you create a strong foundation for an active and satisfying sex life. Small, consistent efforts toward fitness, nutrition, and self-care can lead to greater energy, confidence, and pleasure in your intimate relationships.

CHAPTER 5
Mindfulness and Relaxation Techniques

Mindfulness and relaxation are powerful tools for enhancing intimacy and pleasure, especially as life's stresses and responsibilities grow with age. By focusing on the present moment and cultivating a sense of calm, you can deepen your connection with your partner, heighten sensations, and enjoy a more fulfilling sexual experience.

The Role of Mindfulness in Sexuality

Mindfulness is the practice of being fully present and engaged in the moment, free from distractions or judgment. When applied to intimacy, mindfulness can:

Enhance Sensory Awareness: Heightened attention to touch, sound, and other sensations can make each moment more pleasurable.

Reduce Performance Anxiety: Letting go of self-conscious thoughts allows you to focus on enjoyment rather than outcomes.

Strengthen Emotional Connection: Being fully present with your partner fosters a deeper sense of trust and intimacy.

How to Practice Mindfulness During Intimacy

Focus on your breath to anchor yourself in the present moment.

Pay attention to each sensation—skin-to-skin contact, warmth, or the rhythm of movement.

Let go of distractions or intrusive thoughts by gently redirecting your focus to your partner and the experience.

Relaxation Techniques to Reduce Stress

Stress is a common barrier to intimacy, as it can dampen libido and increase tension. Incorporating relaxation techniques into your routine can improve overall well-being and create the mental space needed for intimacy:

Deep Breathing Exercises

Take slow, deep breaths to calm your nervous system.

Practice synchronized breathing with your partner to build a sense of connection.

Progressive Muscle Relaxation (PMR)

Tense and release different muscle groups to reduce physical tension and increase relaxation.

Meditation

Spend 5-10 minutes a day in quiet meditation, focusing on your breath or a positive intention.

Incorporating Mindfulness into Foreplay and Sex

Mindfulness can transform both foreplay and intercourse into richer experiences:

Set the Mood: Create a relaxing environment with dim lighting, soothing music, or candles to engage your senses.

Slow Down: Take your time exploring each other's bodies without rushing toward climax.

Communicate Through Touch: Use gentle caresses to express affection and explore what feels pleasurable for both of you.

The Power of Sensory Awareness

Mindfulness emphasizes tuning into your body's sensations and responses. By focusing on sensory experiences, you can deepen your pleasure:

Touch: Feel the texture of your partner's skin and the warmth of their body.

Sound: Notice the rhythm of your partner's breathing or the sound of their voice.

Scent: Enhance the experience with subtle fragrances or essential oils.

Practical Exercises to Try
Mindful Touch Exercise:

Spend 5-10 minutes exploring your partner's body with light, deliberate touch. Focus on each stroke and how it feels, without the goal of initiating intercourse.

Body Scan Together:

Lie down with your partner and guide each other through a mental scan of the body, noticing areas of tension and relaxation.

Mindful Eye Contact:

Spend a few moments gazing into each other's eyes, focusing on the connection rather than words or actions.

Mindfulness Beyond the Bedroom
Mindfulness practices outside the bedroom can also enhance intimacy:
Take mindful walks together, paying attention to the sights and sounds around you.

Share gratitude for each other during quiet moments. Engage in yoga or meditation as a couple to strengthen both mental and physical bonds.

By integrating mindfulness and relaxation techniques into your life, you create space for greater awareness, deeper connection, and heightened pleasure. These practices allow you to slow down, savor each moment, and build a more intimate and meaningful relationship.

CHAPTER 6

Spicing Things Up: New Positions and Settings

Variety is the spice of life, and that applies to your intimate moments as well. Introducing new positions and settings can reignite passion, deepen connection, and create exciting experiences for you and your partner. Experimentation doesn't have to be intimidating—it's an opportunity to explore, have fun, and strengthen your bond.

Why Change Matters

Breaking Routine: Familiar routines, while comforting, can sometimes lead to monotony. Trying something new adds excitement and anticipation.

Discovering New Pleasures: Different positions and environments can stimulate areas of the body in unique ways, enhancing pleasure for both partners.

Strengthening Connection: Sharing new experiences fosters trust, communication, and emotional closeness.

Exploring New Positions

Trying new sexual positions doesn't mean you need to perform acrobatics—it's about finding what feels good and works for both of you.

For Greater Intimacy

Spooning: A relaxed and close position, ideal for a slower, more intimate experience.

Face-to-Face Seated: Sit facing each other on a chair or the edge of a bed, allowing for eye contact and gentle touch.

For Deeper Sensation

Modified Missionary: Elevate the hips with a pillow for enhanced angles and deeper penetration.

Doggy Style Variations: Adjust the height or use cushions to find the most comfortable and pleasurable alignment.

For Playfulness and Creativity

Standing Positions: Incorporate furniture or a sturdy surface for support.

Reverse Cowgirl: Adds a playful twist and allows for new sensations and visual appeal.

Changing the Setting

Sometimes, a simple change of scenery can bring a fresh perspective to your intimacy.

Around the House

The Kitchen Counter: Adds spontaneity and excitement.

The Shower: Water can enhance sensuality, but be mindful of safety—use a non-slip mat for stability.

The Living Room: Use the couch, floor, or other furniture to create new experiences.

Outside the Bedroom

Staycations: Book a local hotel for a night to enjoy a change of atmosphere without traveling far.

Vacation Romance: Explore intimacy in a cozy cabin, beachside villa, or anywhere new and inspiring.

Outdoor Adventures (Where Safe and Private)

Picnic blankets under the stars or secluded spots can add an element of adventure and romance.

Incorporating Props and Accessories

Enhance your experience with accessories designed to add variety:

Pillows and Cushions: Support comfort and creativity in different positions.

Sensory Enhancements: Introduce blindfolds, feathers, or massage oils to heighten anticipation and pleasure.

Couples' Toys: Explore devices designed to enhance intimacy together.

Communicating and Collaborating

Experimenting with new positions and settings requires open communication and mutual consent:

Start with a Conversation: Share ideas and preferences with your partner in a relaxed, non-pressured setting.

Be Playful: Treat experimentation as a fun adventure rather than a serious task.

Check-In Often: During intimacy, ask your partner how they feel and adjust as needed.

Tips for Success
Take It Slow

Don't rush into complicated positions or settings. Gradually introduce changes that both partners are comfortable with.

Prioritize Comfort and Safety
Use sturdy furniture and ensure any outdoor settings are private and safe.

Laugh Together

Not every attempt will go perfectly, and that's okay! Embrace the awkward moments and enjoy the process.

Spicing things up is less about perfection and more about connecting in new, exciting ways. By embracing variety, you not only enhance pleasure but also deepen the emotional and physical bond with your partner. Remember, the journey of exploration is just as rewarding as the destination.

CHAPTER 7
When to Seek Professional Help

Sometimes, challenges in intimacy and sexual wellness require the guidance of a professional. Whether it's physical discomfort, emotional disconnection, or unresolved conflicts, seeking help is a proactive step toward enhancing your relationship and overall well-being.

Signs You May Need Professional Support

Physical Issues Impacting Intimacy

Persistent pain during intercourse (for women, this could include vaginal dryness or discomfort; for men, difficulty maintaining an erection or delayed ejaculation).

Loss of libido or inability to achieve orgasm despite stimulation.

Chronic health conditions or medication side effects that interfere with sexual satisfaction.

Emotional or Psychological Barriers

Anxiety, depression, or stress that diminishes your interest or ability to engage in intimacy.

Negative self-image or body confidence issues affecting your comfort during intimacy.

Past trauma, such as sexual abuse or assault, impacting your sexual relationship.

Relationship Struggles

Communication breakdowns around intimacy, leading to misunderstandings or resentment.

Conflicts or unresolved issues causing emotional distance.

Mismatched desires or expectations in the relationship that feel difficult to navigate.

Major Life Changes

Transitioning through menopause, post-partum recovery, or significant health events.

Adjusting to changes in your relationship dynamic, such as becoming empty nesters or coping with a partner's illness.

Types of Professionals to Consider
Medical Professionals

Consult a gynecologist, urologist, or primary care physician for physical concerns such as hormonal imbalances, erectile dysfunction, or vaginal dryness. Seek specialists for chronic conditions (e.g., diabetes, heart disease) that may affect sexual health.

Therapists and Counselors

A sex therapist can help address specific issues around intimacy, performance, or sexual satisfaction. A couples therapist can guide you through communication barriers or relationship conflicts affecting your sexual connection.

An individual therapist may be beneficial for addressing personal barriers like anxiety, trauma, or low self-esteem.

Pelvic Floor Specialists
Physical therapists specializing in pelvic health can assist with issues such as painful intercourse, pelvic pain, or postpartum recovery.

Certified Coaches or Educators
Sexual wellness coaches or educators can offer guidance on techniques, intimacy-building exercises, or tools for spicing up your relationship.

How to Prepare for Seeking Help
Identify the Issue
Reflect on what challenges you're experiencing and how they're affecting your well-being or relationship.

Communicate with Your Partner

If the issue involves your relationship, share your feelings openly and discuss the possibility of seeking help together.

Find the Right Professional

Look for licensed or certified specialists with expertise in the area of concern. Reading reviews or seeking recommendations can help ensure a good fit.

Be Open and Honest

During sessions, share your concerns, experiences, and goals openly. Professionals are trained to create a safe, judgment-free environment.

Benefits of Seeking Professional Help

Improved Understanding: Gain insight into the root causes of challenges and learn effective solutions.

Strengthened Communication: Develop tools to express desires, concerns, and needs more clearly.

Renewed Connection: Rebuild trust and intimacy, deepening your bond with your partner.

Enhanced Sexual Satisfaction: Address physical or emotional barriers to rediscover pleasure and fulfillment.

Seeking professional help is not a sign of failure—it's an act of commitment to yourself, your partner, and your relationship. By addressing challenges head-on with the support of an expert, you can open the door to greater intimacy, understanding, and satisfaction.

CHAPTER 8
Emotional Intimacy and Connection

Physical intimacy thrives when supported by a strong emotional connection. Emotional intimacy—the ability to share your innermost thoughts, feelings, and vulnerabilities with your partner—is the foundation for trust, understanding, and enduring passion. Nurturing this connection can make your relationship more fulfilling and your sexual experiences deeper and more meaningful.

What is Emotional Intimacy?

Emotional intimacy goes beyond physical closeness. It involves:

Open Communication: Sharing your true feelings, dreams, and fears without fear of judgment.

Mutual Understanding: Feeling seen and understood by your partner on a deep level.

Trust and Vulnerability: Being able to express your authentic self, knowing your partner supports you.

Shared Experiences: Building a reservoir of meaningful moments together, from small daily interactions to significant milestones.

Why Emotional Intimacy Enhances Physical Connection

Builds Trust: Feeling emotionally safe with your partner allows you to relax and be fully present during intimate moments.

Deepens Desire: Emotional closeness fosters attraction and strengthens your desire to connect physically.

Heightens Satisfaction: Intimacy becomes more satisfying when underpinned by a deep emotional bond.

Ways to Strengthen Emotional Intimacy

Prioritize Quality Time

Spend uninterrupted time together regularly, whether through date nights, walks, or shared hobbies.

Make an effort to be fully present during these moments, putting aside distractions like phones or work.

Practice Active Listening

Listen to your partner without interrupting, and validate their feelings by acknowledging their emotions.

Use empathetic responses such as, "I understand how you feel," or "That must have been difficult for you."

Express Appreciation

Regularly share what you love and admire about your partner.

Simple affirmations like "I'm grateful for you" or "I love how thoughtful you are" can strengthen your connection.

Be Vulnerable

Open up about your own feelings, even when they're challenging to express.

Share your hopes, fears, and dreams to create a deeper sense of partnership.

Show Physical Affection Outside the Bedroom

Small gestures like holding hands, hugging, or cuddling reinforce emotional closeness and show your partner they're cherished.

Creating Emotional Intimacy During Conflict

Disagreements are a natural part of any relationship, but how you navigate them can either strengthen or weaken emotional intimacy.

Stay Calm

Avoid reacting impulsively or defensively. Take a moment to breathe and collect your thoughts.

Focus on Solutions

Rather than assigning blame, work together to find solutions to the issue at hand.

Apologize and Forgive

Acknowledge when you're wrong and apologize sincerely. Similarly, be willing to forgive and move forward.

Use "I" Statements

Express how you feel without attacking your partner, e.g., "I feel hurt when…" instead of "You always…"

Intimacy-Enhancing Activities

Ask Meaningful Questions

Use prompts to learn more about each other, such as "What's something you've always wanted to try?" or "What's a favorite memory we share?"

Create Rituals Together

Establish small, meaningful habits, like sharing a cup of coffee each morning or having weekly check-ins about your feelings and goals.

Practice Gratitude
Each day, share one thing you're grateful for about your partner. This reinforces positive feelings and appreciation.

Work on Shared Goals
Collaborate on projects or dreams, whether it's planning a trip, starting a hobby, or setting relationship goals.

Emotional Intimacy in the Bedroom
Communicate Desires and Boundaries
Talk openly about what you enjoy and what you'd like to explore, ensuring both partners feel heard and respected.

Focus on Connection, Not Just Performance

Let go of the pressure to perform and focus on being present with your partner, enjoying each other's touch and energy.

Share Afterglow Moments
Spend time cuddling or talking after intimacy to deepen your emotional bond.

The Lifelong Benefits of Emotional Intimacy
Cultivating emotional intimacy enhances every aspect of your relationship, fostering a sense of security, love, and partnership. It helps you weather life's challenges together and keeps your connection strong, ensuring a vibrant and fulfilling relationship at every stage of life.

CHAPTER 9
Exploring Sexual Health Supplements

Sexual health supplements can play a supportive role in enhancing libido, stamina, and overall sexual wellness, especially as age-related changes or lifestyle factors impact intimacy. These supplements, derived from natural ingredients or targeted formulations, are designed to address various aspects of sexual health for both men and women.

Before diving in, it's crucial to understand the benefits, potential risks, and best practices for using supplements safely and effectively.

Common Types of Sexual Health Supplements
For Enhancing Libido

Maca Root: Known as "Peruvian ginseng," maca may boost libido and energy levels.

Tribulus Terrestris: Believed to enhance libido by increasing testosterone production.

Fenugreek: Contains compounds that may increase sexual arousal and desire, especially in women.

For Improving Stamina and Performance
L-Arginine: An amino acid that supports blood flow, potentially enhancing erectile function and sensitivity.
Panax Ginseng: Often used to improve stamina and reduce fatigue, with potential benefits for erectile function.
Horny Goat Weed: Contains icariin, a compound thought to improve blood flow and sexual endurance.

For Balancing Hormones
Ashwagandha: An adaptogen that may help regulate stress hormones and improve libido.
DHEA (Dehydroepiandrosterone): A hormone precursor that may support libido and energy, especially during menopause or andropause.

For Enhancing Pleasure

Ginkgo Biloba: Promotes better circulation, potentially heightening sensation and arousal.

Zinc: Plays a role in testosterone production and reproductive health.

Supplements for Women's Sexual Health
Black Cohosh

Commonly used to alleviate menopausal symptoms, it may also enhance libido by addressing hormonal imbalances.

Evening Primrose Oil

Supports hormonal health and may help with vaginal dryness.

Vitamin E

Improves skin elasticity and moisture, which can benefit vaginal tissue health.

Supplements for Men's Sexual Health

Saw Palmetto

May support prostate health and balance testosterone levels.

Yohimbe

Derived from the bark of an African tree, this supplement has been used to enhance erectile function and stamina.

Nitric Oxide Boosters

Supplements like beetroot powder or L-citrulline support blood flow, essential for healthy erections.

Safety and Considerations

Consult Your Doctor

Always consult a healthcare provider before starting any supplement, especially if you're on medication or have health conditions such as hypertension, diabetes, or heart disease.

Research Quality and Purity

Choose reputable brands that provide third-party testing and transparency about ingredients.

Watch for Side Effects

Natural doesn't always mean safe. Be aware of potential side effects such as allergic reactions, digestive discomfort, or interactions with medications.

Follow Recommended Dosages

Taking more than the recommended dose doesn't guarantee better results and could lead to adverse effects.

Lifestyle Changes to Enhance Supplement Benefits

Supplements work best when combined with a healthy lifestyle:

Stay Active: Regular exercise improves circulation and boosts libido.

Eat a Balanced Diet: Nutrient-rich foods support hormonal balance and energy levels.

Manage Stress: High stress levels can dampen libido and hinder sexual performance.

Get Enough Sleep: Quality sleep is essential for hormone regulation and overall vitality.

Myths and Realities
Supplements are Not a Quick Fix

While supplements can provide support, they are most effective as part of a holistic approach to health.

Not All Supplements Work for Everyone
Individual results can vary based on factors like age, lifestyle, and underlying health conditions.

Beware of Overhyped Claims
Be cautious of products that promise instant results or claim to cure sexual dysfunction completely.

When to Consider Supplements
Experiencing a gradual decline in libido or stamina due to aging or stress.

Seeking natural support during menopause, andropause, or hormonal changes.
Addressing specific concerns like circulation, energy, or hormonal balance.

Sexual health supplements can enhance intimacy and pleasure when used thoughtfully and safely. With the right approach and guidance, these tools can help you reclaim vitality and enjoy a more fulfilling sexual relationship at any age.

CHAPTER 10
Conclusion

Continuing to Explore and Enjoy Your Sexuality After 40

Sexuality is a lifelong journey that evolves and deepens with age. Reaching your 40s doesn't signal the end of passion; in fact, it can be an exciting new chapter of self-discovery, intimacy, and connection. With the right mindset, communication, and tools, you can continue to explore and enjoy your sexuality in meaningful ways.

Embrace the Changes

As we age, our bodies change, but that doesn't mean our sexual experiences have to become less fulfilling. Understanding these changes—whether physical, emotional, or psychological—helps you adapt and find new ways to connect with yourself and your partner. Whether it's exploring new positions, embracing mindfulness, or seeking professional advice when needed, every step you take in nurturing your sexual health contributes to a deeper, richer connection.

Nurture Emotional Intimacy

Physical intimacy and pleasure are enriched when emotional intimacy is prioritized. As you move through your 40s and beyond, deepen your emotional bond with your partner through communication, shared experiences, and vulnerability. A strong emotional foundation fosters trust, safety, and connection, making intimacy more fulfilling.

Explore New Possibilities

There's no limit to how you can keep things exciting. Trying new positions, settings, or even introducing sexual health supplements can spice up your relationship. Experimenting with new ideas doesn't require drastic changes but a willingness to explore and communicate with your partner. These little shifts can reignite passion and bring fresh energy into your relationship.

Invest in Your Health and Well-being

Taking care of your physical and mental health is essential for maintaining a fulfilling sex life. Regular exercise, healthy nutrition, mindfulness, and stress management are all key components to feeling good both inside and out. When your body feels well, your mind feels at ease, and intimacy becomes more enjoyable.

Seek Help When Needed

If challenges arise—whether physical, emotional, or relational—don't hesitate to seek professional support. A healthcare provider, therapist, or sexual wellness expert can help guide you through any obstacles and offer solutions tailored to your needs. Seeking help is not a sign of weakness but a proactive step toward enjoying your sexual health and well-being.

Celebrate Your Sexuality

Sexuality doesn't have an expiration date. In fact, your 40s and beyond can be some of the most fulfilling years of your sexual journey. Embrace this time of growth, exploration, and joy. Celebrate the connection with yourself and your partner, knowing that pleasure, intimacy, and joy are always within reach.

As you continue to grow, remember that your sexual well-being is a dynamic part of your life that deserves attention, care, and exploration. With the right tools, communication, and self-awareness, you can keep your sexuality vibrant and fulfilling for years to come.